HOW TO LOOK GOOD ALWAYS:

BE YOUR STUNNING SELF

SUSAN RUSSELL

Copyright @2022Dr.Hill Levine

All right reserved

TABLE OF CONTENTS

INTRODUCTION

Can we just be real for a minute: when we look great, we feel much better (as well as the other way around). The craving to need to look great consistently is in no way, shape or form shallow. In the event that we don't feel much better about what we look like, we will be unable to go about as the best version of ourselves.

Regardless of what our identity is, what we do, and what we're chipping away at, everyone needs to know how to look great.

We should admit that our general public is focused on our looks, and despite the fact that we see a lot of ravishing assortment recently, there's as yet a steady strain to look great wherever you go.

What's more, frankly, I don't believe it's something terrible. Knowing how to look great can open a lot of opportunity for you, it can assist you with winning the hearts of those you like and it might assist you with making a superior profession. It's appalling, however it is valid, and you can exploit it. Significantly more - you can truly flourish in your life (regardless of your age!), utilizing your self-esteem, taking care of oneself, and self-esteem to underline and improve your normal excellence. Remember that beauty is many times in the eyes and ears of the beholder, and there is in every case more going on than might be expected!

Yet, before we plunge into how to look beautiful always, we should examine in the event that it's importance first!

CHAPTER ONE

HOW IMPORTANT IS LOOKING GOOD EVERY DAY?

The solution to this question relies upon you. At the point when I'm honest with myself, I realize I perform better at work on days that I feel good about my looks, regardless of whether I'm working from home! I'm likewise confident in my relationships when I feel beautiful.

Looking great regularly frees us up to potential open doors and conceivable outcomes. Research shows that individuals who look great are more effective. Maybe it's the additional certainty you get from looking great. Or on the other hand perhaps people are simply more responsive to other people who have invested energy and exertion into their appearance.

While it might appear to be insignificant, we can confront real challenges when we don't invest energy into our appearance. We might act less confidently around others because we feel self-conscious.

To top it all off, we could pass up amazing open doors we in any case would have hopped on assuming we had felt better about ourselves and our looks. So, considering that, be straightforward with yourself about how important looking great every day is to you.

WHAT IT MEANS TO LOOK GOOD?

To look good means, you're looking your very best - healthy, blissful, pretty, and put together.

Its vital to know that to look good doesn't mean you need to follow some sort of unambiguous beauty standard or attempt to seem to be your favorite Instagram model. You don't have to be perfect.

Knowing how to look great is more about learning a couple of fundamental style and beauty rules that can make anyone stand out. It's tied in with underlining your remarkable features, your character, and the manner in which you see your general surroundings. It's vital to take note of that when you look great and feel appealing, your whole life is impacted in a good manner.

This is the way to look great, boost your attractiveness and make every little thing about you extremely magnetizing!

HOW THE PRESSURE TO ALWAYS LOOK GOOD CAN BE STRESSFUL

Obviously, the strain of sorting out some way to constantly look great can cause pressure by its own doing. As ladies, we're continually barraged with promotions for various cosmetics items, costly skincare schedules, and extravagance spa therapies. For some ladies, the strain of looking good always can simply be an excessive amount to deal with.

The beauty industry endeavors to let us know we're not enough. Our normal hair variety isn't adequate, we should have a perfectly measured proportion of body hair (in precisely perfect spots), and our nails ought not be seen except if they're newly manicured. These messages are unsafe, and they're false.

We don't need to spend a fortune, lose hours of our long stretches of time, or go through difficult treatment to look great, and we unquestionably don't require beauty marketers to let us know how to look beautiful every day!

We can look lovely impeccably normally by doing basic, reasonable activities. These activities will assist us with looking great, and they'll assist us with feeling significantly better, as well.

CHAPTER TWO

WHY YOU DON'T HAVE TO SPEND A FORTUNE TO LOOK GOOD EVERYDAY

You put your best self forward when you're cheerful, healthy, and put together, and you unquestionably don't have to keep a particular stunner guideline or look a specific method for looking great. You will normally look great when you feel far better.

On the off chance that you're battling with your mental health, concealing your unhappiness with makeup can be troublesome. What's more, attempting to do so can be harmful. All things being equal, making the moves to cause yourself to be in a better mood can address the genuine purposes behind your misery is the most effective way to push ahead and normally look great.

In like manner, you don't need to change your body shape or totally reset your closet to look great. At the point when you accentuate your uniqueness and show off parts that cause you to feel beautiful, you'll naturally look good.

CHAPTER THREE

TOP TIPS ON HOW TO ALWAYS LOOK GOOD

Anyway, would you say you are considering how to look good regularly without going through hours before the mirror or dropping many dollars on cosmetics? Looking great regularly doesn't mean you need to invest long stretches of additional energy on your appearance.

It additionally doesn't mean you need to buy new items or pay for services that would only make you feel good temporarily. These tips will show you how to always look great with little time and effort.

1. Maintain great cleanliness

This one might sound senseless, however maintaining great cleanliness is particularly significant in our post-pandemic world. While a significant number of us changed to working from home (to some degree briefly), we might have understood that nobody would see on the off chance that we didn't shower each and every day.

Be that as it may, you can't misjudge the usefulness of an everyday shower. Regardless of whether you went through the day working from your couch, a speedy 5-minute shower will help you look and feel new and clean. What's more, on the off chance that you don't wash your hair consistently, a fast spritz of dry cleanser can leave you feeling revived and non-oily.

Additionally, your dry shampoo might try and furnish you with some additional volume and sparkle! Maintaining great cleanliness is the way I look good regularly without burning through much cash.

2. Iron your outfits

The contrast between badly creased garments and pressed garments is dumbfounding. A badly crumpled outfit can cause it to seem like you just rolled out of bed. A newly pressed one, be that as it may, can make you look cleaned and set up. Assuming you end up hurrying out the door each day, take five minutes the prior night to iron tomorrows outfit. You'll be so happy you did!

Similarly, now is the ideal time to change out the sweatpants, regardless of whether you're working from home. Wearing night robe or sweatpants during the business day might have felt fun - in any event, daring - for those first few weeks of social distancing. However, wearing warm up pants every day of the week can remove the enthusiasm from your step.

In the event that you totally can't stomach the sweatpants, take a stab at matching a cute set of tights with a comfortable sweater! A casual yet chic outfit is the manner by which I look great regularly while working from home.

3. Follow a skincare routine

Glowing skin is an extraordinary method for looking good always! Furthermore, you needn't bother with the best in class line of skincare items from your number one retail chain to accomplish glowing skin. All things being equal, make a moderate skincare routine utilizing essential, dermatologist-recommended items.

You may just need a cleanser, a lotion, and some sunscreen for a decent skincare routine. In the event that you're battling flaws or your skin is extra dry or oily, you may likewise need to use a toner, serum, or medication to accomplish the glowing skin you need! The main thing is to be consistent and give your skin the normal treatment it deserves.

4. Use cosmetics decisively

Having a mark cosmetics look is one more tip for how to look good every day! In this way, assuming you're a young lady who loves cosmetics, make a cosmetics routine that features your best elements.

Assuming you're focused on looking good every day, you don't have to go overboard with cosmetics. Similarly, likewise with your skincare routine, focus on finding a moderate cosmetics routine that features your best elements naturally.

Toning it down would be ideal while you're adjusting your cosmetics routine while attempting to set aside time and cash. Find essential items that don't take you over 10 minutes to apply every morning.

For instance, you may just need a good foundation, concealer, bronzer, blush, one shade of eye shadow, mascara, and one lipstick or lip gloss for a final pop of color! You'll be out the door in the blink of an eye.

5. Smile often, smile wide!

Allow your magnificent whites to radiate through. A few examinations have shown that more stronger smiles bring about additional appealing countenances. Significantly more effectively, smiling can really encourage you too!

Assuming you're feeling down, take a stab at smiling at someone else or simply all alone in the event that you're without anyone else. Despite the fact that it might feel senseless, a certified smile can lift your mind-set and improve your attractive features.

6. Shop more efficiently

Wearing well-made clothes that fit your body type is a simple method for looking good. However, clothing can likewise be perhaps one of the costliest thing in your budget! The key is to shop more efficiently. It's completely conceivable to look great while keeping a moderate closet.

Focus on finding pleasant apparel that is made to last and buying classic basics you can mix and match with different pieces in your closet. Keeping away from fast fashion might be ideal.

In any case, clothing bought from fast design producers can quickly go out of style and doesn't last very long anyway. Being fashionable on a budget is the means by which to look great regularly without burning through every last cent!

7. Get a hair style that is not difficult to style

Assuming that you have a hair style that requires 30 minutes or more to style every day, you might battle to look and feel good on a consistent basis! For those mornings you simply have to get out the door, a classic, simple to-keep up with hair style is your best friend. Numerous hair styles just require a fast fixing or refreshing with the hair curler - and they look perfect!

So, assuming that you're struggling with your hair each day, the issue may not be your hair. It very well may be your hair style! Examine different choices with your hairstylist next time you see her - or track down another hairstylist in the event that you're consistently getting bad styles. Having a tasteful hairdo is the manner by which to continuously look great!

8. Take control of your body language
Non-verbal communication says a ton regarding how we feel, and it can likewise improve how we look. You can undoubtedly further develop how you look by focusing on your stance and your body languages. Sitting upright makes you look

more confident, while slouching over can make you look inadvertently insecure.

Furthermore, keeping your arms uncrossed and in a vacant position can make you look really inviting and responsive to other people, as could a smile and a proper measure of eye at any point contact. Focusing on your non-verbal communication is a simple method for making yourself immediately look great.

9. Remain hydrated

Drinking sufficient water is fundamental for looking great regularly! I can't exaggerate this. At the point when you're hydrated, your skin is better. Drinking sufficient water can assist you with having battle wrinkles, kill skin break out, and decline tingling from dry skin.

You'll likewise see upgrades in your appearance and pore size when your lovely skin is hydrated. Remaining hydrated is a sound way how to continuously look great.

10. Find your signature perfume

… how to look great with little effort! In all honesty, a decent and fitting fragrance is your straightway to that.

An intriguing, sexy, or unique smell can say a ton regarding your character and make an attractive air around you. Smelling lovely is incredibly appealing and you should simply track down that one aroma that accommodates your character, style (and nose!) impeccably.

Try not to flood yourself with an expanse of scent however - a couple spritzes on your neck or hair are sufficient and you'll blow some people's minds without a doubt. Toning it down would be best when you need to look great because less is always more when you want to look good!

12. Eat well and work out

A healthy way of life can assist you with building a fit and alluring body, which is without a doubt… However it can likewise assist you with fighting social confidence issues, nervousness, and stress over-burden. At the point when you feel quite a bit better, you look great, so remember the significance of enhancing your internal world too. Working out, taking care of oneself, eating new leafy foods (they're brimming with nutrients!), journaling and contemplation are astounding ways of keeping your inward beauty sparkling. You can likewise get massages to further improve circulation and loosen up tense muscles (or brain!).

One more significant method for really focusing on your wellbeing and beauty is to take high-quality supplements. Fundamental nutrients, amino acids, and minerals are essential for each cycle in your body: hair development, skin recharging, nail keratinization - and so on! Our tissues are "hungry" for supplements. In the event that you don't get enough of them in your eating routine (honestly, it's hard!), consider high-quality supplements.

With regards to hair, skin, and nail wellbeing, likely the most famous enhancement decisions are Biotin and Collagen. These important supplements assist your skin with remaining flexible, support quicker hair development, keep your skin flaw free, and perform various tasks to keep you looking perfect. You can find Biotin and Collagen supplements in powder form, container form, or fluid form, which has the most elevated bioavailability. A good example of superior grade, fluid Biotin + Collagen supplement is Wellabs Fluid Collagen for hair development.

13. Use sunscreen

Shield your beautiful skin from hurtful UV beams by wearing sunscreen consistently. Sunscreen keeps your skin sound and liberated from untimely maturing, and it likewise shields you from skin disease. It can go about as an additional moisture boost also! Finding a lotion or foundation with sunscreen is a simple method for safeguarding your beautiful face without adding an additional move toward your daily schedule.

You could likewise have the option to trade out your ordinary body cream with a salve that contains sunscreen. Make a point to utilize SPF 30 or above. In sunnier months, you might need to expand your SPF for much more security.

You can constantly look great notwithstanding your financial plan!

14. Know your value

To wrap things up - to look great, work on remembering your value as well. Cherishing and valuing yourself doesn't mean you need to be presumptuous, or loaded with yourself.

Knowing your value, feeling certain about your capacities, embracing your qualities and life manages essentially shows the world that:

You like yourself;

You realize that you look great;

You don't actually tend to think about what every other person thinks.

That is called confidence and that is compellingly provocative!

Now you know how to look great always regardless of your budget! Looking great every day is simple when you feel good. Doing things that cause you to feel good and that are great for your body will normally bring about you looking great, so center around making little steps like the ones depicted above to do right by you consistently quickly.

It isn't important to invest a great deal of energy or money to look great consistently. As a matter of fact, investing more energy or money on your appearance can really cause you stress you needn't bother with, which could degrade your endeavors to look lovely!

Keep in mind, you can look great consistently by taking little, straightforward activities like pressing your garments, putting on sunscreen, working on your stance, and flaunting your lovely grin.

CHAPTER FOUR

HOW TO LOOK GOOD AT WORK

Have you at any point contemplated whether there is anything specific that helps you to look good at work? There is!

A few things can assist you with raising your looks thoroughly in a business or commercial environment and even assist you with performing better.

1. Ensure your nails are immaculate

I prefer not to say it, however it's not difficult to get threatening looks on the grounds that your nail clean is chipped. On the off chance that you're a representative, a faultless nail treatment is an unquestionable necessity. In addition to the fact that it helps you to look great while connecting with others, but at the same time it's stylishly satisfying to your own eyes.

I understand you're occupied enough with all that work over-load, so my proposal is to pick gel nail treatment, which can endure much longer than regular polish. A decent gel manicure will last you as long as 14 days! Do it once and forget for two weeks, girl – now that's life!

In the event that you don't have time or assets to visit a nail salon two times every month, put resources into an at-home gel polish unit. Trust me, you will save many dollars over the long haul.

2. Remain Hydrated

This might sound interesting, however if you need to take a gander at work, you must remain hydrated. People underestimate the significance of water time and again! Absence of moisture can make your face look drained and dull - this can be all kept away from with a sip of water a few times each hour. You don't have to chug an entire gallon - simply ensure your body is getting customary water ingestions, and you'll look great since you'll be appropriately hydrated.

 3. Dominate in power colors

Have you at any point saw how striking high contrast, or red outfits look? Something about these varieties make you look great and practically mesmerizing when you wear them.

So when you endeavor to take a gander at work, wear garments in colors that talk: power, confidence, status, energy! Profound dark, snow white, cherry red, and naval force blue are great! Furthermore, these tones look very smart in chilly cold weather months, similar to December. Heels, a smidgen of excellent scent, red lipstick are different choices that assist you with looking great and expert.

CHAPTER FIVE

HOW TO LOOK GOOD IN PICTURES

Ok, the camera game! Knowing how to look great in pictures is a really helpful thing to learn, so here are my best tips that I'm certain you will cherish.

1. Take your photographs from far away

The number 1 example to learn to look great in pictures is to make distance. Taking pictures very close generally makes your face look twisted and absolutely not what you resemble actually. To look great in a photograph, ask another person to snap it for you (a couple of feet separated), or timer function and pose!

2. Never take your photos from the base

Snapping a picture from the base point makes you look unusual and adds extra "weight" that doesn't necessarily exist truly. Then again, taking pictures from the top point of view underscores your eyes and cheekbones, which will constantly look great, in any photograph.

3. Play with points

All of us has a point that suit us - you simply need to know yours! That's what to do, don't hesitate for even a moment to experiment and take a lot of pictures just to figure out which point looks the most complimenting (and no, it's not senseless or shallow). When you find it, play it like your best card and stress your best side to look great in each selfie (and life, obviously!).

CHAPTER SIX

HOW TO LOOK GOOD WITHOUT MAKEUP

Cosmetics is amazing, however there are times in our lives when we simply need to look great… without it. Perhaps your working environment has strict no cosmetics rules, perhaps you're welcome to a third date with that person you're pounding on truly hard, or perhaps you simply don't have any desire to overpower your generally drained skin.

There are such countless motivations to look great without cosmetics and fortunately, it isn't so difficult!

1. Take the best skincare you can afford right now

SPF sunscreen, bb cream, covers - spoil your skin so it tends to be glowing, healthy, and delicate with practically no cosmetics on. Dealing with your skin doesn't need a ton of exertion, yet it can compensate you with an even composition and sound pores. Assuming you battle to find what truly suits your skin, see your dermatologist - this way you will try not to overspend on items that don't help your skin. Likewise, now and then our skin needs more grounded medicines to cut down aggravation, dispose of microbes, or limit scars and kinks.

2. Appreciate messy haircut's

Hello, to look great while you're all natural, it's likewise the best chance to partake in those messy, straight-from-the-bed hairstyles! Basically wash your hair and let it air dry. On the off chance that you don't like how your hair dries, do it right (or better) by adding delicate, messy waves or straightening those frizzy bad boys with a flat iron.

3. Keep them lips delicious!

At the point when your skin is clear, and your hair looks perfect, the last thing to check for is your lips. Are they being spotless? Are they being moisturized?

To make your lips look good (and overwhelming) without cosmetics, put them on a decent lip scrub session.

Then, apply a liberal amount of lip balm and check on them a couple of times each day to ensure they actually look great!

CAN YOU LOOK GOOD AT ANY AGE?

Totally, 100 percent yes! Since you're accustomed to seeing more youthful models wherever on the media, it doesn't imply that only young ladies can look great.

There are lots of ladies who look great in spite of their age - and that is not a special case for the standard of some sort. A couple of instances of ladies who look great after 50 (or even 80!) are Christie Brinkley, Demi Moore, Jennifer Lopez, Halle Berry, Elizabeth Hurley - this list could go on and on.

You can age gracefully and look good at the same time - everything boils down to your decision and the manner in which you feel about yourself in any case.

To look great, you really want to deal with your appearance - that is certain. In any case, have you seen that many of these focuses are aimed at your self-love, confidence, and self-esteem? Since hello, even the prettiest girl can look great taking cover behind four walls - yet does it matter on the off chance that she's hesitant to show her beauty to the world?..

Confidence and courage to embrace the manner in which you look are obviously the absolute most significant things to recall when you need to look great. It can make individuals succumb to you, and not on the grounds that you're pretty… This is on the grounds that you like yourself and that is totally, incredibly, attractively appealing.

CONCLUSION

These are the quickest and simplest ways of being pretty, cleaned, confident, and overpoweringly appealing any place you go. Dealing with your looks is likewise an extraordinary type of taking care of oneself, since it supports your confidence assists you with cherishing yourself more, and works on your mind-set. You could endeavor to be pretty even while you're staying at home, since there is no difference either way.

Obviously, you are wonderful and alluring as of now, however I can't envision anybody appearing the same after following all of these straightforward methods. So if you have any desire to figure out how to be pretty even on your most exceedingly terrible days, these straightforward methods will assist you with upgrading your look without obtrusive strategies or costly salon visits. Nothing shouts "pretty!" in excess of a lady who just loves herself and won't hesitate to play with her style, cosmetics, and non-verbal communication… You may not be even mindful of how much feminine power you hold!

Lastly… If you can and need to upgrade your looks - you have 100 percent right to make it happen, however much you need, regardless of what any other person is talking about.